12 PRACTICAL NATURAL REMEDIES, FOR AN IMMEDIATE RELIEF FROM COMMON DISORDERS

A handbook based on the work
"Star bene con poco"
(Staying healthy with little)

DR. MARIO FRUSI

DEDICATION

I am dedicating this book to all those asking me to only feel good once again, without being interested into knowing why my prescriptions will be effective

CONTENTS

ACKNOWLEDGMENTS

I thank all those who supported me, believing in my approach towards healing, one which is completely person-focused, instead of illness-based

PREMISE

"At that precise moment, I understood that the fragility of the person who had called upon me in search of a solution to his problem would not have allowed him to discuss the causes of her illness with me. He was only interested into healing, immediately."

The declared intent with which I wrote my second book, "Star bene con poco", was to provide the reader with a series of practical remedies, for treating the most common diseases; these are the ones which won't kill, but alas, may also significantly compromise a patient's life quality.

Later on I decided to also provide a multimedia e-book along with the paper work, in order to make the information contained in the book more easily usable, through footage aimed at enriching the text with a sensory audio-visual experience.

On the other hand, this handbook intends to satisfy readers searching for further summarizing: the issues addressed in this work are covered in a more complete manner in "Star bene con poco", yet in this book, they are seen from the point of view of many of my patients, who were simply looking for a practical, immediate and natural solution. One that is effective for their problems.

Indeed, I had already written my previous book with particular attention towards those who required my help, almost as if I was a mechanic who has to fix a car, highlighting those exquisitely practical paragraphs in bold. Yet, the work that follows is the extreme synthesis of what I previously released.

I decided to devote myself to it when I realized that, as a doctor, it is also worth for me to acquire the ability to pass on to the patient only information which is strictly needed for making him or her feel good, and that my ambition to involve him in understanding the causes and implications of his illness essentially only satisfies a personal desire of mine, one which very few are willing to grant me.

Therefore, this book is born based on the assumption that modern society has us all used to having "everything, immediately", without even needing to understand the reason for a given treatment's effectiveness, and that a doctor, like any other technician, should simply provide a solution to a problem, and quickly.

So this is why I'm giving you your "health manual", which you may also consult easily, with the first part dedicated to illustrating all the chapters in which the suffered illness is discussed.

Perhaps you already figured out for yourself, this approach is not at all the one I prefer to work with, but my professional ethic gives priority to your well-being, over any other consideration.

In order to fully enjoy the benefits of the remedies suggested in this book, I'm inviting you to fully identify yourself with the severity of your illness, before experimenting with the techniques described in this work.

My wish is that what follows below may prove useful also for you, as it was for the many patients I had the pleasure to personally meet.

Dr. Mario Frusi

Cuneo, Italy - November 10th, 2019

PART 1

A REMEDY FOR ALL KINDS OF AILMENTS

In this first part, I will address, in a specific and separate way, 12 of the most common ailments for modern man. For each and every one of them, I will offer you a simple and natural remedy which you may try for yourself, in complete autonomy. This work tries to combine simplicity with practicality, but if the description given in the handbook was to prove insufficient for your needs, you may read about it in a more extensive way on my book "Star bene con poco", or rather, you may buy the digital version, complete with audio-video material which is useful for a deeper understanding of the techniques.

ANXIETY CAN GO AWAY BY BREATHING

Anxiety is that feeling of emptiness in the center of the chest, due to less pressure in the thoracic space above the diaphragm, something we experienced for the first time at birth when the lungs initially expanded.

Therefore, and quite surprisingly, the psychological state of anxiety directly originates from a physiological condition of low pressure, and as such, can be solved with a simple mechanical movement which compensates for this situation: a sort of embrace exercised by the lungs on the heart interrupts the signal to the brain of that feeling of physical discomfort, which we usually interpret as anxiety.

Indeed, "breathing a sigh of relief" doesn't refer inhaling, but instead means to exhale the old air already present in the lungs. This is precisely what forces us to do this exercise.

This also explains the relaxing effect of cigarettes: indeed, the most calming part of the smoking act is the one after inhaling the smoke, not the absorption of all the toxic substances in the blood.

Thus, anxiety can be overcome very simply, by using a sequence of actions one can perform even without anyone noticing:

- choose a position in which the spine is aligned;
- empty your chest by blowing in a gentle, moderate and constant manner, stopping only when emptying it more would require a lot of effort;
- wait to breathe in for a moment before feeling the lack of air (maybe ten seconds if you are at rest);
- let the air in gently and without forcing it, only up to the quantity the lungs are comfortable with, and trying not to let the will intervene;
- take a break and, if you haven't yet reached a state of well-being, repeat the exercise.

ANGUISH CAN BE EXTINGUISHED BY JUST BLOWING

A situation of sudden stress can trigger a state of anxiety far more disabling than the general distress described in the previous chapter, which therefore would need to be faced with a much more energetic breathing technique, more similar to the ventilation produced by a bellows. Eventually, you can go on until a significant improvement in the general conditions can be felt.

You can repeat this exercise even in a few series of 10 for improving mental concentration or promoting sleep, but you'll always have to practice it with caution, the same one needed when you dose your medicines: if the muscular effort needed for the exercise is unbalanced, you may experience an aching neck, headaches, dizziness, a high heartbeat and even a lower-back contraction!

I have to specify that, with "generalized muscle contraction", I intend the contraction of all voluntary muscles (including those of the face with the mandibles tightening "individually", meaning without pressing the dental arches one against the other) stiffening completely, but without movement, in order to not dislocate the spine: the back will not arch, shoulders and head won't move, and even if hands and feet were to also twist slightly, the movement wouldn't rebound towards the knee or the elbow anyway.

This will have the effect of reducing adrenaline in the blood, forcing it from the muscles to the lungs, and of reducing general muscular response to physiological values; it will also exert a symbolic catharsis effect, by allowing you to "hunt down the fear demon".

But let's get to the exercise:
- lying on a soft surface, help yourself into aligning your back by bending your knees and using a modest rise under your nape;
- inhale by taking in a lot of air, but keeping the body soft and stopping before the shoulders

become stiff (this is the sign indicating that you reached your maximum lung capacity);
- hold the air for 2-4 seconds in the lungs (not less, in order to avoid getting drunk on oxygen);
- exhale all the air with a puff which, in a couple of seconds, becomes progressively more intense up to its maximum, and at the same time exerts a "generalized muscle contraction" (this effort must be done while blowing to avoid a potentially dangerous increase in pressure inside the body);
- when your lungs are almost empty, stop blowing and loosen your muscles;
- if you don't yet experience a feeling of breathlessness, stay with your chest empty for at least a couple of seconds;
- still keeping yourself loose, you can now start the cycle again.

TUMMY ACHES CAN GO AWAY
WITH MANIPULATION

All pains deep in the bowels located in the area between sternum and pelvis (from abdominal indigestion-related pain, to menstrual aches or constipation, rather than the discomfort caused by a calculus), have a counterpart on the surface: it is a subcutaneous fibrousness which represents them and supports them. If the latter is reabsorbed with careful and wise manipulation, followed by the anti-inflammatory action of an arnica montana cream (don't use its macerated oil!), the internal pain will also disappear.

The manipulation described below can be used as needed in an emergency, but if the pain recurs frequently, it is advisable to plan an intervention on a weekly basis, until all tissue inhomogeneities are completely reabsorbed.

The idea is to perform a "pinching and chalking" manipulation, individually working on all the points below which a disorder is perceived: a consistent fold of both skin and subcutaneous tissue must be grasped between the thumb and the index/middle finger, rubbing the fingertips between them so that the tissues pinched between the fingers go into friction.

You will feel the pain due to the mechanical gesture, but also the connection between the subcutaneous manipulation and the movement of something deep within the symptom area. You will therefore have to insist for a few minutes on each point, until you clearly feel a qualitative and quantitative improvement within.

In case of particularly abundant subcutaneous tissue, it is useful to stiffen the abdominal wall, almost like with an intention to raise your legs with your knees extended, in order to isolate the area to work on. This way, you will operate on the underlying tonic plane, which the muscular contraction makes perceptible to the touch, but not on the internal viscera, with a slightly different technique: dry, with an important and rotary manipulation (or rebounding), or with the help of a gel, using your finger knuckles or an instrument like a large marker pen with very rounded edges.

Take your time and manipulate slowly and deeply, avoiding acceleration, in order to work on the "knolls" typically present where a problem manifests in depth: these bloated parts are the densities on which you'll have to insist.

Don't be discouraged by the annoyance that this manipulation can cause in case of an acute event: after a while, a clear sensation of "pleasant pain which is actually good for you" will take over.

A FLOATED BELLY WILL GO AWAY WITH A HERBAL TEA

The problem of meteorism (also called "bloated belly") afflicts in different measure our entire population, and as such, it can't be defined as a disease, but as an annoying consequence of altered intestinal fermentation, which already begins with the colic development of the infant.

The intestinal gas, normally generated in a few small bubbles, should be reabsorbed by the mucosa, and by being transported by the blood, should return to the atmosphere through the lungs.

Unfortunately, though, quality and quantity of ingested food, an insufficient bowel movement or even regular seasonal alternation, can induce the micro-organisms which produce it to excessive fermentation, with consequent swelling and, at times, even pain.

Notwithstanding the fact that it's always advisable to take care of developing a healthy bacterial flora, also by using some good probiotics, the remedy illustrated below has the most modest goal of solving the disorder's disturbing symptomatology, but also of avoiding all those inconveniences caused by gas pressure, which by pressing on the diaphragm, ends up influencing what's above, causing anxiety and arrhythmias.

I suggest you a herbal tea, excellent to sip at the end of a meal: boil a spoonful of the following preparation for a couple of minutes, filter it and drink it hot.

Fennel regulates intestinal motility and promotes bubbles breaking down, licorice is a sweetener and a gastro-protector, while mint has proved to be a good antispasmodic.

The doses for the preparation are:

- 50 gr. Fennel seeds (these are fruits, botanically!);

- 40 gr. Ground root licorice;

- 10 gr. Peppermint leaves.

A FLU GOES AWAY WITH REST, DECOCTS AND CANDIES

Cold and flu are disorders of viral origin, facilitated by colder winter temperatures. You can effectively face by simply letting them do their natural course, while just staying at home.

This, besides avoiding an increased contagion risk for the community, allows you to indulge the outbreak of fever without antipyretics: the rise in body temperature triggers a beneficial sweating which expels toxins, counteracts the virus's replication and... gives you an altered state of consciousness capable of bringing yourself to the same level of awareness given by a shamanic concoction!

So, if you are not particularly young or very old, I advise you to allow your body temperature to rise even of a couple of degrees, and instead concentrate on limiting symptoms, most importantly that annoying sense of occlusion in the airways.

As a basic intervention, I invite you to drink a filtered decoction obtained from two or three minutes of infusion "with lid" (after a minute in boiling), several times a day and very hot:

- Triturated root licorice, a heaping spoon;
- Chili pepper, a pinch;
- Sage, two dried leaves;
- Cinnamon, a stick of a couple of centimeters;
- Juniper, 5-6 berries;
- Cloves, 1-2.

If well tolerated, the vasodilating action of a spoon of hard liquor, to be mixed together with the preparation, will favor the general medicinal effect.

You can guarantee yourself some immediate relief, with frequent repeatability, also through the decongestant effect on the mucous membranes of nose and throat exercised by the balsamic principles contained in many kinds of drops (available in pharmacies, parapharmacies or herbal shops, and strictly to be applied in the nostrils facing upwards) and candies (with mint, without sugar, to be slowly dissolved in the mouth, avoiding the latter in case of poor sensitivity to swallowing); but don't forget to integrate with potassium and magnesium, because the loss of salts is very common during episodes of fever, sweating and physical fatigue in general.

Furthermore, apart from recommending you a fresh vegetables-rich diet, due to their high content of water-soluble vitamins and antioxidant substances, I'd recommend you to wash your nostrils frequently.

This involves mechanically removing the flu virus when it still stagnates in the oro-pharyngeal mucosa, introducing warm salt water into a nostril, and then letting it flow out of the other nostril and/or from the mouth, and ending with some salt water gargle. Repeating the wash every 4/5 hours will prevent the virus from ending up in your bloodstream.

A NECK PAIN WILL FADE AWAY WITH AN EXERCISE

The rebalancing of unbalanced tensions is always a valid tool for getting your full health back, even when there are no obvious manifestations of stiffening and pain in a given muscle band, as in the case of neck pains, when the contraction affects the oblique profile which extends precisely to the base of the neck.

In this chapter we will precisely address this annoying disorder, with an exercise capable of re-calibrating the degree of muscle tone through which information is passed to the brain, by neuro-muscular spindles.

Sitting on a comfortable chair with your back well attached to the backrest and your forearms on the armrests, let your rear neck gradually stretch by tilting your head forward, slowing down the fall, to the point of not perceiving pain, but a tolerable pulling.

In this position, you must complete 3 complete breathing cycles, as follows:

- take a deep inhale, but keep your shoulders soft;
- hold the air in for a few moments without stiffening any part of your body;
- exhale with a resounding "sigh of relief", until your airflow of air empties spontaneously.

During the exhalations you may feel your head tilting more forward, but also a pleasant sense of stretching of your muscles up to the lower back, due to the fact that the muscles of the entire spine are functionally connected to each other.

Now, while still leaving your neck immobile (i.e. with the head tilted forward), you have to slide slowly on the chair, so as to bring your pelvis towards the front edge of the seat surface. At the end of this movement, you'll find yourself with your trunk tilted backwards, and your head forward.

Now, keeping your shoulders soft, lift your head up as if to look in front of you and complete the exercise, bringing the chest upright without lifting the chair, but helping yourself with your hands and forearms and coordinating the lifting effort with the expiration (you can move your chest by squeezing the armrests or grasping, with your hands positioned like pliers, a table which you previously positioned in front of the chair).

YOUR BACK CAN BE UNLOCKED BY EXTENDING IT

Stretching the lumbar region requires more effort than the one needed for the neck in the previous chapter, as the musculature is more pronounced and powerful in this region.

The following exercise, to be carried out on the bed before falling asleep or in all cases on a comfortable surface (a blanket or a carpet), requires delicacy and extreme slowness, both in carrying it out and in getting up (turning on one side and helping yourself with your arms).

With your upper limbs, progressively lie down on the ground with your knees softly bent and your head slightly raised by a pillow.

One after the other, bring both knees to the chest as much as possible using your muscles only at the beginning of the movement, then grab them with the corresponding hand and finally hug them with your forearm, in a gentle, patient and constant traction effort. Do this while always remembering that you are performing a fine work of quality and inner perception, not an athletic gesture.

After achieving the smallest angle between thighs and trunk that you can tolerate without discomfort, keep this position for three long and slow sighs: a good inhaling depth, a pause with a filled chest, a completely passive emptying phase and another pause with your chest emptied. If you experience a tightening of the neck, reduce the amount of inhaled air and/or the impetus with which you inhale it.

After completing your three sighs, release the knees in reverse order compared to how you grabbed them, then return control to the leg muscles.

CERVICAL AND SCIATICA PAIN WILL GO AWAY WITH CHILLI PEPPER

The "supporting contraction" in the high trapezium profile area is a simple consequence of the bipedal posture, which by bearing weight on only two limbs, can literally be said to "stay up with their shoulders". A tension at this level, when not directly perceivable, can at least be triggered by pressure or stapling.

Yet, muscle stiffness tends to worsen in a vicious circle, because the muscle fibers compacted by the contraction prevent oxygen and nutrients supplies towards the muscle itself.

Thus, the solution consists in gently applying a formulation on the high trapezoid, containing a good dose of red pepper or its active ingredient, capsaicin, in order to reactivate the blood circulation following the reaction to heat and local redness.

Identify the area precisely and spread a small amount of product, using a sheet of crumpled kitchen paper to avoid touching it with your fingers. It would however be preferable to find someone to help you, because the painful cord sits "behind" the trapezium you see in the mirror.

Since you won't be able to predetermine skin sensitivity, in order not to risk burns or an overdose (the active ingredient penetrates very easily into the skin but is difficult to remove, even with oil and cleansing milk), observe the first modest application after fifteen minutes, and if you haven't experienced significant reactions, repeat it by rubbing a little more.

Otherwise, if redness appeared but the spasmodic painful contracture did not loosen, then it's time to also work on the musculature running alongside the dorsal spine, applying the chili pepper formulation, first in the more rigid areas between the inner margins of the shoulder blades, and then at the neck.

You can use this medicinal repeatedly and as needed, while also taking into consideration a potential, yet highly unlikely, risk of allergy.

As a reference, two or three treatments a day can

however generally be continued, for a week without risks or fears of damage.

The same pepper formula can also be used when pain occurs in the lower part of the chest: a lumbago, a sciatica, a stiffening of a buttock or along a lower limb.

The application must begin on the lumbar paravertebral muscles, and if necessary, continue on the muscular mass inside the buttock and on the compact cord (often rigid), which extends horizontally about four fingers below the iliac crest.

It is interesting to note that this method can give appreciable results also on the unconscious tensions appearing on the muscular apparatus, in a little localizable way, and which tend to self-preserve themselves, as they're not conscious: the application of an ointment can represent a rapid exit from an existential torment you have been suffering from for a long time, but also a new lease on life, for living it with more enthusiasm, free from the heavy burden of your experiences.

A HALLUX VALGUS CAN HEAL SPONTANEOUSLY ONLY BY UNDERSTANDING ITS CAUSE

In this chapter, I will convince you that hallux valgus is a disease which is not inherited genetically, but learned at a behavioral level, very often as a consequence of a male-dominated and self-destructive social pattern, which finds it right for daughters to suffer like their mothers.

In fact the genetic foundation for this deformity is practically null, with the big toe becoming instead deformed as a result of a postural attitude, defined by British osteopathy as "widow's hump", that the female child learns from her mother (or even her grandmother): an ancestor, hit by a particularly serious existential occurrence, will assume a posture which will make her look "crushed by the weight of what happened to her", one with her neck inclined forward, and the big toe compensating the consequent muscular overload on the whole organism caused by the head thrust, by distorting itself.

Ergo, a daughter will never inherit such deformity through genes, but will conform to a behavioral "fatigue" pattern, recreating it in her own body.

By personally verifying this truth, through the exercise that I'm offering you, will entice you to work on the emotional matrix of your muscular tensions, obtaining results which are not only limited to this pathology.

After standing at attention for at least ten seconds, push your neck and head forward, holding the rest of the body as it was. In a few minutes it will be easy for you to feel a sensation inside the forefoot, right next to the big toe: something between annoyance and pulling, which soon turns into an overload of weight and tension.

This shows you how the big toe region is stimulated by incorrect head posture, and you can now easily imagine that the deformity is a simple consequence of a compensation attempt, and as such, can regress just through postural exercises.

INTOXICATIONS CAN BE CURED WITH A ENEMA

Caffeine, present in coffee and tea, besides being a good antispasmodic for the bronchial tract, has important antioxidant effects, capable of restoring the metabolic circuits of the liver when the anti-poisonous action of the latter is compromised, by the excessive quantity of toxic waste produced by a disease, which ends up engulfing it.

However, this medicinal activity brings a risk damage potentially produced by carcinogens developed during roasting and especially, those resulting from the cardiac excitement triggered by the consumption of several cups of coffee.

German oncologist Gerson had already identified a way to separate the caffeine's benefits from its damages, taking his coffee through an enema instead of orally: in this way the drink is absorbed directly by the colon, and so conveyed to the liver by the portal vein, without damaging other organs and tissues. Here it also performs choleretic (bile producing) and antispasmodic actions locally, even without the risk of a biliary colic in kidney stones sufferers.

This detoxifying practice, repeated with regularity, proves very useful for reversing the toxins accumulation symptoms of many diseases, and over time, the diseases themselves; but it is also a healthy hygienic action, also of great help both after a simple indigestion and as a good habit, useful for ensuring optimal well-being. The indications are simple.

Prepare 2 coffeemakers worth 6 coffees cups, or alternatively, a less common 12-cup moka coffeemaker, then add cold water to the total quantity of 1 liter of liquid.

Fill the edema with the preparation at a warm temperature.

Then hold the liquid for at least 12 minutes, so that all circulating blood passes three times into the colon and comes into contact with the water-soluble coffee substances, first of all the caffeine, which in this atypical assumption, will not reach the brain.

If any spasms make it difficult to hold the liquid in

your intestine for so long, you can proceed with an enema filled with only warm water (300-400 ml) held back a few tens of seconds, before the coffee. In any case, repeating the treatment over time will always make it easier to reach the recommended 12 minutes.

THE OVERWEIGHT FACES WITH THE KETOGENIC DIET

An overweight organism suffers both an aesthetic and a health damage: indeed, it is known that a lean body benefits from a greater harmony, and diseases related to obesity (psychic, metabolic, cardiovascular pathologies, and cancer) seem to be the bio-logical restitution of the damage resulting from having maintained a nutritional attitude which has departed from its basic parameters.

Given that an ideal weight can be easily maintained by adopting a plant-based diet, the ketogenic diet is a modern shock therapy which owes its name to the ketone bodies, of which it stimulates production, when it forces the body to consume adipose tissue, by depriving it of sugars.

In fact, it exploits the life-saving mechanism which was very useful to our ancestors, when with no available sugars, they sustained themselves with the reserves present in their bodies.

Moreover, the ketones circulating in the blood gave them, and give us today, some valid tools for surviving in a situation of emergency (which was very much real in former times of famine, and is only sought today): good humor, lack of appetite and mental lucidity.

So excluding sugar and carbohydrates in general from your diet, in favor of protein food, while still guaranteeing an adequate supply of vitamins and minerals, you can safely simulate this beneficial "sugar famine", and reshape your body to a perfect condition, while gaining back your health.

PART 2

REMEDIES WHICH WILL MAKE ALL ILLNESS GO AWAY

In this second part I will tell you about three tools already available to you, useful for living without getting ill, or at least for minimizing your chances of getting ill.

This is real prevention, as I will teach you a lifestyle which completely prevents the development of diseases, instead of adapting the term "prevention" to the early diagnosis of existing diseases, as is usually done when we talk about screening.

Through the use of the three tools I will describe

in detail, you will really be able to do a lot for your health, and in complete autonomy.

This is the truth, within certain limits, even in front of an already overt pathology, because the body naturally tends to restore its state of natural health, and therefore the same attitude that prevents it from losing it in advance is also able to create the conditions for favor it, giving the body many ways to get well again.

It's so much simpler than you think.

POSTURAL REALIGNMENT GYMNASTICS

A good mechanical structure in the body will provide a significant contribution for healing from many diseases, and the same postural re-education path, in search of a new tensional order between all parts, allows for a progressive awareness for stress-structural loads management, and since our musculature is the seat of emotions, it promotes access to the depth of one's own existential roots, with the opportunity for a profound inner change.

In conclusion, a good tensional adjustment of chest, neck and limbs, by performing the proposed exercises with frequent and patient repetitions, promotes the body's correct way of maintaining its health, from both a physical and psychological point of view.

At a microscopic level, the proposed exercises tend

to defibrotize musculature invalidated by the human body's energy-saving system: an unused muscle progressively replaces its contractile and extensible fibers with a connective tissue of coriaceous, fibrous texture. Once the fibrosis is triggered, the muscle is functionally no longer a muscle.

However, this involution process is reversible, and even just 10 minutes of postural exercises can trigger the ever-so needed reconstructive mechanisms: the stimulus re-synthesizes acto-myosin molecules, which are able to contract the muscle, and myoglobin molecules, which act as precious oxygen stocks for these tissues.

Furthermore, a change in tenso-structure also involves a virtuous modification of the cerebral neurological network: like a tree's roots will extend towards water and nourishment, yet withdrawing from the sterile soil, neuroplasticity intends for new extensions to always develop near an interconnection which has proved useful. Indeed, intelligence means by definition "capacity for connection".

UPPER BODY STRETCHING

This exercise combines cervical and lumbar

stretching in a single progression of movements, with the patient gradually stretching his paravertebral muscles downwards.

Despite being a clearly complete sequence, and therefore proving useful in preventive terms for the important postural realignment it provides, this exercise can also be used as a "first aid" to achieve immediate relief, in case of episodes of acute pain.

Sit in a chair with your belt unfastened, then try to bend the different regions of your spine forward, starting from the neck, until you find your head between your legs, slightly apart, facilitated in this slow movement by your arms's weight.

In this final position you have to sigh three times, obviously limited by your chest's compression, then go up in a sequence perfectly mirroring the earlier descent, absolutely avoiding to activate your neck musculature, but helping yourself first with your forearms on your thighs, then raising up with your hands on your knees.

Finally, slowly slide on the chair bringing your pelvis towards the front edge of the seat surface, closing the exercise as if you were stretching your neck alone.

DOMESTIC MANIPULATION

This exercise reduces stiffness building up in your muscles when performing physically demanding tasks, or after being subjected to psychic tension.

Unlike the other ones you can't do it alone, but you'll need a "manipulator" that follows the instructions below.

First the manipulator will have to identify those points on which to intervene subsequently, through a modulated pressure, exerted with the fingertips on the two muscular "salami" on the sides of the vertebral column, rising from the pelvis up to where the neck begins: these are the points where there's the most hardness to the touch, or where you report resistance or even pain.

Then the action begins on these points, always starting from the bottom: exerting a modest pressure with the index finger, which must be kept firm without rubbing, a soft rotation movement of the wrist will begin, drawing a cone in the air with its vertex being the fingertip leaned on the surface.

Your manipulator will have to increase pressure as long as he perceives a collapse of superficial muscular layers, after which he'll pass on to the next phase, concluding the action with three vigorous pinches first.

Indeed, this gesture intervenes on the local contracture, first resolving the lack of blood with a polite and growing pressure, and then completing the work with the vasodilator effect of pinching.

Once at the neck, he or she will proceed from the center outwards in the high trapezoid, moving almost to its upper edge.

This micro-massage, defined as "Far East", induces a beneficial relax even in the performer.

THE GROUND EXTENSION EXERCISE

The exercise of stretching to the ground, especially if practiced with daily regularity at the same time of day, gives an extraordinary feeling of well-being. This is a consequence of the body's self-expansion (exclusively longitudinal in man, on three axes in an amoeba's body!) which confirms the bi-directionality of a universal concept in the animal world: fear and suffering contract us, while self-esteem and prosperity will stretch us.

Lying on a blanket, under which you will have placed a couple of books as a nape support (in order to create a uniformly rigidity bed), place your arms at 30-50° away from your chest, with the palms of your hands turned towards up. Take care to smooth out the cavity which will have most likely formed at the lumbar level between your body and the floor, progressively resting on the ground, starting from the pelvis area, as if unrolling a rug.

Now modulate a breath, without prior inspiration but with the air you already have in your lungs, as if you wanted to animate the flame of a candle, placed at 20-30 cm. away in front of you, with a simultaneous contraction of your abdominal (flattening towards the ground) and buttock muscles (in retention). You need to leave all other muscles relaxed, possibly even the pelvic and perineum ones, yet only preventing your knees from falling sideways.

Once the total and natural emptying of your lungs is reached, let air passively in by opening your mouth, and at the same time loosening buttock and abdominal tension.

Once passive lung expansion is exhausted, regain control to maintain a short phase (a few seconds) of soft stillness in the chest, which will have self-filled.

Repeat the cycle, returning to blow and contract

the musculature, for a total of 10 minutes.

Then move on to the second part of the exercise, which consists in 5 minutes of long and deep "sighs of relief", and finally get up again by turning first on your side.

Once you master this sequence of actions, you will introduce some beneficial work with your neck, while making sure that the added movement is not transmitted to the lower back, causing lumbar buckling. In the pause, raise your neck a little, like if you wanted to "look upwards" (considering that we are in a lying position, this means shifting our gaze to the wall farthest from our feet), so when you start exhaling/contracting, flatten the neck and get yourself a bit of a double chin, with a feeling neck stretching (with an excursion and intensity effort similar to that needed for looking at a bookshelf in front of you, from a plane above your eyes four to five floors below).

THE SEATED POSITION EXERCISE

This exercise also involves the previous "ground stretching", and I'd suggest to perform it for just 3 minutes after the 10+5 minutes during which you lay down. It involves different postural dynamics, in fact only introducing the work needed to support you, carried out by your core muscles.

Sitting as far forward as possible (almost without resting your thighs) on a stool or a rigid chair, oscillate until you get the perception of a having your chest as vertically flat as possible, with its weight resting symmetrically on the two pelvic bones within the gluteal mass.

Contracting abdominals and buttocks, then blow some air through your mouth with a neck movement bringing your gaze from where the wall in front of you meets the ceiling, down until it's horizontally flat.

Follow with some spontaneous inhalation, holding your neck steady, and then start the cycle again by blowing and contracting, while looking upwards.

THE STANDING POSITION EXERCISE

As soon as you feel ready, you should definitely add 3 more minutes of the same exercise, but this time in a standing position, for completing a daily activity requiring a total of about twenty minutes.

Standing exercises will rectify your lumbar spine (pelvis rotation pivoting on the hips, so that the pubic bone is pushed upwards and the sacrum downwards; keeping the knees slightly bent, perhaps with the help of your hands), for the rest you will repeat the sequence exactly as when you were lying on the ground or sitting.

During the final exhaling phase, you should perceive this perfect spine axialization: it is only a subjective tensional datum, far from reflecting a real geometric straightening, but it is nevertheless a useful perception for the defibrotizing reshuffling underway in your body.

ENGAGING THE ILEO-PSOAS

The ileo-psoas is a powerful muscle lodging in the depth of our chest, and is capable of conditioning much of the activity.

You can easily engage it with a small variation of the seated position exercise: for the whole exhaling time, while contracting and progressively lowering your gaze, add some feet pressure towards the floor, with a significant yet not massive effort.

You will feel a sensation of strength, despite the gesture's lack of effectiveness while seated.

ADDING THE ARMS

Still for complementing the seated exercise, you can now add one arm's movement: with your hand near the shoulder and the palm facing forward with semi-bent fingers, use the exhale time to get your elbow to be almost tense (in order to not engage the shoulder) in a muscular effort of "pushing yet holding at the same time", running an imaginary stretched steel wire through the hollow between thumb and forefinger.

Then complete the path backwards during passive inspiratory expansion.

On the next cycle you will obviously change hand, alternating the initial hand, until you gain the coordination needed to move them both together: one forward and one backward.

ADDING THE LEGS

You have to introduce a step which, repeated and alternated on your legs, becomes a smooth and homogeneous rectilinear walk (although always in an resistance effort), which allows to not practice sitting and standing exercises anymore, but to go from lying to full, maintaining a total commitment of 20 minutes.

Start by sort of "sitting on a bench in the air", advancing the left foot of a few centimeters, and by keeping the load on your right side, lowering the expiratory buttock. Then "stand up" for the next exhalation. Repeat the cycle a few times, then change sides.

Add the hand rocker effect now, moving with the latter along with the foot and positioning the other close to the armpit from the "sitting" side.

Then transform the seat into a step, shifting the weight on the front foot and starting the translation, in a sequence similar to Tai Chi.

I can however acknowledge that it's impossible to explain to you such a complex movement in words, so this is why I provided many explanatory videos with the book from which this handbook is taken, "Star bene con poco".

FRUITARIAN NON-OXIDATIVE FOOD

The most currently validated theory for explaining decay in organisms is based on the concept of "oxidation": the chemical reactions necessary for the life and cells development require, as a biological price, the accumulation of oxidized radicals. It seems that the degree of wear and tear of an entire body can be assessed precisely based on the progressively accumulated amount of "rust", until the degenerative process interrupts the vital flow.

To counteract oxidation, you have two tools available which involve a re-evaluation of your eating habits:

- you need to take sufficient amounts of antioxidants, through supplements or foods which contain them (especially fresh vegetables, although to a lesser extent, they are present in eggs and milk);

- it is important to consciously reduce the total quantity of food that you consume daily, while stopping to have it symbolically represent a lack of existential nutrition.

In principle, in order to prevent your body from succumbing, engulfed by the waste products of cellular metabolism, you can run your body's engine at a lower rev number, "by pressing less on the accelerator", meaning by introducing less fuel, or by adding some additives to this fuel so that it burns with less harmful consequences.

Well, there is a diet with a very low caloric content and extremely healthy for the antioxidants it provides: practically put, it produces little waste, and at the same time, reduces the damage caused by it. Going back to the automotive comparison, it allows you to travel with very little fuel and burn what little you consume.

It is the fruitarian diet, which expects you to eat only fruit in the broadest botanical sense of the term: the sweet fruit that we all know, fruit vegetables (pumpkins, courgettes, tomatoes, peppers, cucumbers... which are technically fruits because they come from a flower!) and fat fruit (avocado and olives).

As far as my lack of my awareness goes for scientific demonstrations attesting the biological parameters of those who feed only on fruit, the fruitarian diet seems sustainable in the long term, and while adopting it myself without too much rigor, I have ascertained its indisputable benefits: typical feverish "flu" syndromes decreased in number, intensity and duration, my usual neck-shoulder rigidity was significantly reduced, and I also noticed a lower reactivity to insect bites.

In fact, all this can be traced to the reduction of silent inflammation present in the organism, probably triggered by the human habit to feed on "a bit of everything", while all other advanced apes are almost exclusively fruit-eating.

Indeed, "postprandial leukocytosis", a general alarm in the blood and tissues with consequent activation of an immune protection through the mobilization of a large number of white blood cells, does not occur when the ingested food consists exclusively of fruit and other raw vegetables. This suggests that everything you habitually introduce into your body, and particularly cooked food, is interpreted by the latter as a potential threat, one to defend itself from.

In particular, besides a generic reduced caloric intake, fruit contains very little protein. On average they are found in the same order of magnitude as those present in breast milk, a perfect food for the infant, which however, still has to shape a large part of its body. Otherwise, the diet you are used to also contains ten times as much of them, and requires your body to dispose of the waste that comes with it.

Further confirming the fact that man is a fruitarian, also other data converge: the stature, grip and size of our hands, our sight, teeth, moderate gastric acidity, intestines length... in all probability, our ancestors used to eat as we still do today, but only due to reduced fruit availability, to be attributable to glaciations or perhaps as a result of the nomadic initiative which led them to move away from the central African area from which they originated.

Getting to feed on fruit alone, through a progressively more and more depriving food degrowth, means to restore the power for which your body has been designed: a nutritional reconversion, desirable in healthy and ecological terms, which if stimulated by the Government, would have a favorable impact as much on public health budgets as on pollution from intensive farming.

Afterwards, I will show you the food scheme that I followed with personal satisfaction, and which I consider to be introductory and therefore adequate for this text. It leaves freedom in your choice of fruits, giving however correct indications on the intake of sugary foods during the working day, when the body needs energy.

BREAKFAST: from 2 to 4 apples, to satiety;

LUNCH: sweet fruit, free choice in quality and quantity;

DINNER: prevalence of fruit, vegetable, some sweet fruit to taste.

CONTROLLING OUR BODILY PH

During the degradation of foods to their basic components, waste materials are produced with a predominantly acidic chemical connotation, which leads to general unhealthy body acidification, at both an intercellular and intracellular level.

In order to establish how acidifying a given food is, the concept of PRAL (Potential Renal Acid Load) has been defined, which quantifies its effect at urinary level: a high PRAL food will produce a marked change in urine, which will tend to be acidic. The usefulness of this parameter is linked to the fact that an acidic food may not be so for the body (as in the case of lemon), and vice versa, (for example mozzarella).

In general, acidifying foods are meats, cheeses, simple sugars and spirits, while almost all vegetables are alkalizing.

The importance of this lies in the fact that research shows how an acidifying diet worsens sports performance, reduces cognitive abilities, exacerbates disturbing physical and mental sensations, induces asthma crises, worsens menstrual pain, and aggravates bone health and damage from chronic diseases.

In order to empirically convince yourself of how much nutrition affects your body pH (the alkalinity degree) recorded through urine, don't hesitate to buy a pack of "urinary pH test strips" at your pharmacy, wet one with your urine and compare the color you took with the scale from 5 to 8 shown on the package. Repeat the check regularly and adjust your diet, aiming to keep yourself at a pH between 6.5 and 7.

www.ingramcontent.com/pod-product-compliance
Lightning Source LLC
Chambersburg PA
CBHW071019260726
48662CB00022B/790